Healthy Diet For Healthy Lifestyle

How to control your diet by choosing what food is good for your health, and enjoy a healthy lifestyle.

By

Linda M. King

Disclaimer

If you purchase this book without a cover or purchase a PDF, JPG, or spat copy of it, it is intelligently taken property or a phony. In light of everything, neither the makers, the wholesaler, nor any of their laborers or experts have gotten any portion of the copy. Besides, misrepresenting is a known street to financial assistance for facilitated bad behavior and mental aggressor social events. We request that you not buy any such copies and report any event of someone offering such copies to Plata Appropriating LLC.

This dispersion is planned to give talented and reliable information concerning the subject covered. Anyway, it is sold with the cognizance that the maker and merchant have not taken part in conveying authentic, money-related, or other master counsel. Guidelines and practices now and again vary starting with one state then onto the next and country to country, and if legal or other expert assistance is required, the organization of a specialist should be searched for. The essayist and wholesaler unequivocally disavow any liability that is brought about by the usage or utilization of the things in this book.

Presentation

Do you imagine that you want to visit a medical clinic before you carry on with a sound way of life? The response is NO!

I can let you know that what you consume consistently will figure out what sort of way of life you live, either a solid or undesirable way of life. Try not to be frightened, I'm not saying that food is awful, but rather a few food sources are not great for your well-being.

Hi everybody! I go by Linda M. King, I'm 67 years of age, from Dallas

I don't want to take quite a bit of your time since I'm very time-cognizant, so every substance in this digital book will be momentarily made sense of.

Growing up as a food tech understudy assisted me with understanding the great harm that what we admit can cause to our well-being.

Once in a while you don't have to change your primary care physician, your clinic, or the pills you take, you just have to change the food that you're such a great amount in adoration with.

According to there's an idiom that, "Exclusive's food is one more man's toxic substance" There are a few food varieties you want to stay away from for some time or even completely.

We as a whole realize that food is vital to each living thing on the planet, yet the main thing is to know what precisely to eat.

I've been taking as much time as necessary to show individuals around me how to practice good eating habits and carry on with a solid way of life, yet that by itself isn't sufficient to contact a huge number of individuals and assist them with profiting from what I've been imparting to individuals around me in the city of Dallas.

The quickest way I can contact you is to make this digital book, so I educate you to get a duplicate concerning this book for you and advantage of it with your loved ones.

The people who are sending me their declarations today are the individuals who made the move to a solid way of life by paying attention to what I showed them and made the move to rectifying their eating regimens, today am contacting you through this digital book, so utilize the buy button to get a duplicate of this book for yourself.

Disclaimer
Presentation
Chapter One
What is quality food?
The most ideal way to guarantee you're eating strongly is to eat a wide range of sorts of food are the accompanying:
A few instances of calorie-thick and supplement-thick food sources include:
Chapter Two
What Is Infection?
How does Illness Kill?
For what reason do infections happen?
What makes an illness lethal?
What's the deadliest illness?
How would you get away from illness?
Chapter Three
How food can beat sickness in our body framework
The most effective method to involve food as medication to forestall, and invert ongoing sicknesses
Food varieties that help your safe framework
Food sources to stay away from to feel your best
Chapter Four
What food means for wellbeing

Major foodborne sicknesses and causes
Things to be familiar with food illness
What are the 7 significant foodborne sicknesses?
How might you forestall foodborne sickness?
How are foodborne ailments treated?

Summary

Chapter One

What is quality food?

A solid eating regimen is an eating routine that keeps up with and works on generally speaking well-being. A sound eating routine gives the body fundamental supplements, liquid, macronutrients like protein, macronutrients like nutrients, and satisfactory fiber and food energy.

In another manner: A sound eating regimen is great and gives you every one of the supplements you want to remain solid, feel good, and have a lot of energy.

Another Definition: Eating a sound eating routine isn't about severe impediments, remaining ridiculously dainty, or denying yourself of the food sources you love. Rather, it's tied in with feeling

perfect, having more energy, working on your well-being, and helping your temperament.

The most ideal way to guarantee you're eating strongly is to eat a wide range of sorts of food are the accompanying:

1, Have vegetables, salad, or natural products with each feast - they are loaded with nutrients, minerals, and fiber that are great for your well-being, assist you with feeling full, and shield you from ongoing infections. Eat different varieties for the best blend of defensive supplements. Something like five servings of vegetables, salad, and organic products are suggested for a solid eating regimen.

2, Cereals, rice, pasta, potatoes, and breads are extraordinary wellsprings of energy. It's ideal to eat wholegrain renditions of these as they contain fiber to keep your stomach-related framework functioning admirably. The amount you want relies upon your age, size, orientation, and movement levels.

3, Milk, yogurt, and cheddar give calcium and protein. Calcium is required for solid bones throughout life. Pick diminished fat or low-fat assortments, these give a similar measure of calcium and different supplements with fewer calories and soaked fat.

4, Your body needs protein to help develop and keep a sound body, requires consistency as well. Meat, poultry, fish, eggs, beans, and nuts are great ways of getting protein in your eating routine.

5, While getting ready meat dishes, go for lean meats and poultry. Have fish no less than two times per week - white fish on one day and slick fish on another. Slick fish gives fundamental omega-3 fats that keep your heart solid.

6, Beans and eggs are great decisions for sans-meat days.

7, Solid fats are a fundamental piece of a reasonable eating routine yet are just required in tiny sums. Low-fat spreads and vegetable oils, for example, rapeseed and olive oil are ideal. Immersed fats, found in hard fats like margarine, can raise your cholesterol levels.

8, Have sound tidbits like natural products, vegetables, low-fat dairy, and high-fiber oats rather than snacks high in fat, sugar, and salt like desserts, cakes, and crisps. Investigate a portion of our sound nibble thoughts.

9, It's not difficult to fail to remember that beverages make up a major piece of our eating regimens. Water and milk are the best choices, and sweet beverages are the best to stay away from.

Assortment is the key. Your body needs loads of various supplements to remain sound - any food or nutrition type can give every one of these. You don't need to get the equilibrium right at each dinner: attempt to adjust throughout the day or even the week.
Food arranging can assist you with seeing what you're eating and pursuing better decisions than you can make under tension.

The inquiries I generally go over:

1, **What is the significance of a solid eating regimen?**

The significance of a solid eating regimen can't be underscored enough for a sound way of life. A sound way of life can be achieved by keeping a solid eating routine and keeping through every one of the fundamental supplements expected by the body. A legitimate eating regimen plan assists with accomplishing ideal body weight and decreases the gamble of constant sicknesses like diabetes, cardiovascular and different kinds of malignant growth.

2, **Does good food influence our body?**
Quality food gives our bodies the "data" and materials they need to appropriately work. On the off chance that we don't get the right data, our metabolic cycles endure, and our well-being declines.

Assuming we get an excessive amount of food, or food that gives our bodies some unacceptable directions, we can become overweight, undernourished, and in danger of the advancement

of sicknesses and conditions, like joint pain, diabetes, and heart illnesses. So, what we eat is key to our well-being. Think about that considering Webster's meaning of medication: "The science and workmanship managing the upkeep of wellbeing and the anticipation, lightening, or fix of infection.

3, Does quality food influence our cerebrum?

Eating great food that contains heaps of nutrients, minerals, and cancer-prevention agents sustains the cerebrum and safeguards it from oxidative pressure. There is an immediate connection between the food varieties we eat and the working of our minds.

Legitimate, sound nourishment can help the mind in more than one way. A sound eating routine can expand the creation of new neurons, an interaction called neurogenesis. What we eat can likewise influence the synaptic versatility of the mind.

4, How does good food prompt a solid life?

An even eating routine gives you all of the energy you want to keep dynamic over the day, supplements you want for development and fix, assisting you with remaining solid and sound and with forestalling diet-related diseases, like a few malignant growths.

Proof recommends routinely practicing good eating habits, even feasts add to supported weight upkeep, a superior state of mind, expanded energy levels, positive motivation to other people, and the potential for an uplifted personal satisfaction.

Good dieting influences how you feel day to day: A decent eating routine can assist with expanding your energy level, lessen your gamble of heftiness, further develop your muscle strength, and even form more grounded bones and teeth.

5, What sound eating routine has the most calories?

Solid unhealthy food varieties incorporate granola, meats, tofu, fish, avocados, milk, beans, yams, entire grains, and nuts. By and large, the everyday worth (DV) for calories is 2000 calories each day, however, individuals dynamic with strength preparation or different activities might need to consume more.

A few instances of calorie-thick and supplement-thick food sources include:

1, Avocados.
2, Salmon and other slick fish.
3, Nuts and seeds.
4, Full-fat dairy items like yogurt, and milk, and 5, Cheddar.
6, Red meat.
7, Egg yolks.
8, Pork slashes.

6, What solid eating routine kills testosterone?
What you eat and don't eat can hugely affect your well-being, including the chemicals your body delivers and uses.

Research has found that food and in general eating regimen appear to straightforwardly affect chemical creation because your body utilizes different supplements to deliver chemicals like testosterone.

All in all, what food varieties kill testosterone?

Research has found countless food varieties that kill testosterone, yet the main one is Soy

Some exploration shows that consistently eating soy items like tofu, soy milk, and miso might cause a drop in testosterone levels.

One little investigation of 35 men found that drinking soy protein disengage for over 50 days brought about diminished testosterone levels.

Soy food sources are likewise high in phytoestrogens, plant-based substances that copy the impacts of estrogen in the body and change estrogen levels — possibly decreasing degrees of testosterone.

Besides the fact that more exploration expected to is comprehend the impacts of phytoestrogens, however, other examinations have likewise found

clashing outcomes, recommending that soy-based food sources might not affect testosterone levels.
An enormous survey of 15 examinations found that soy food sources didn't influence testosterone levels in men.

7, What food gives energy?
The best fuel for practice is carbs, ideally "complex" ones like organic products, vegetables, and entire grains. Sound fats from fish, nuts, vegetable oils, and avocados can assist with energizing

high-intensity games like significant distance running. Protein can assist with helping an insusceptible framework worn out by work out, nuts and seeds are probably the best food varieties to beat weariness and battle hunger, getting different nuts and seeds in your eating routine can give you solid supplements and energy.
Eating crude, unsalted variants is suggested

Chapter Two

What Is Infection?

Infection is a problem of construction or capability in a human, creature, or plant, particularly one that has a known reason and an unmistakable gathering of side effects, signs, or physical changes.
On the other hand: Infection is any condition that breaks down the typical working of parts of the body, like cells, tissues, and organs.

How does Illness Kill?

Once in a while, they kill cells and tissues by and large. Once in a while, they create poisons that can deaden, obliterate cells' metabolic hardware, or encourage a monstrous safe response that is itself harmful.
In some cases, microorganisms duplicate so quickly that they swarm out and have tissues and upset typical capability.

For what reason do infections happen?

Illness flare-ups are generally brought about by contamination, sent from one individual to the next contact, creature-to-individual contact, or from the climate or different media. Flare-ups may likewise happen following openness to synthetics or radioactive materials. For instance, Minamata infection is brought about by openness to mercury.

What makes an illness lethal?

Once in a while microorganisms duplicate so quickly that they swarm out have tissues and disturb typical capability. Now and again they kill cells and tissues altogether. At times they create poisons that can incapacitate, obliterate cells' metabolic hardware, or hasten a monstrous safe response that is itself harmful.

Numerous infection-causing microorganisms produce poisons and strong synthetics that harm cells and make you sick. Different microorganisms

can straightforwardly attack and harm tissues. A few contaminations brought about by microscopic organisms incorporate Strep throat.

What's the deadliest illness?

Ischemic coronary illness is the main source of death all over the planet. Different circumstances, like stroke, COPD, lower respiratory diseases, and respiratory malignant growths, additionally represent a huge part of passings every year, computer-aided design happens when the veins that supply blood to the heart become restricted. Untreated computer-aided design can prompt chest torment, cardiovascular breakdown, and arrhythmias.
Computer-aided design is responsible for 16% of the world's all-out passings.

How would you get away from illness?

1. Go with quality food decisions
For good well-being and illness anticipation, stay away from super-handled food varieties and eat custom-made dinners arranged with fundamental fixings.

A review distributed in 2019 reasoned that utilization of multiple servings of super-handled food was related to a 62% expanded danger for all-purpose mortality. For each extra serving, all-caused mortality expanded to 18%. These food varieties can cause ongoing irritation, and a typical real interaction can turn out badly which can add to coronary illness, diabetes, and even malignant growth.

Super-handled food includes:
Chips.
White bread.
Doughnuts.
Treats.

Granola or protein bars.
Breakfast cereals.
Moment cereal.
Espresso flavors.
Pop.
Milkshakes.

It's urgent to peruse food marks cautiously, most food varieties that arrive in a bundle have more than five fixings or have fixings that you can't articulate. Numerous food varieties marked as diet, sound, without sugar, or sans fat can be terrible for you.

What do all solid weight control plans share?
They comprise foods grown from the ground, beans, lentils, entire grains like quinoa, earthy colored rice, steel-cut oats, nuts and seeds, and sound oils like extra-virgin olive oil.

2. Have your cholesterol looked at

While checking your cholesterol, your experimental outcomes will show your cholesterol levels in milligrams per deciliter. It's significant to have your cholesterol looked at because your primary care physician will want to encourage you on the most

proficient method to keep up with sound levels, which thusly brings down your possibility of getting coronary illness and stroke.

3. Watch your circulatory strain

Do you have hypertension? Regardless of whether you suspect as much, continue to peruse. Because of information distributed by the Place for Infectious Prevention and Avoidance (CDC), around 45% of grown-ups in the US have hypertension characterized as systolic pulse, or diastolic circulatory strain, or are taking drugs for hypertension.
Ordinary circulatory strain is characterized as pulse <120/80 mmHg. Having hypertension jeopardizes you for coronary illness and stroke, which are driving reasons for death in the US.

Indeed, even little weight reduction can help oversee or forestall hypertension in numerous overweight individuals, as per the American Heart Affiliation.

4. Get up and get rolling

Discard any normal confusion about practicing like that it must be in an exercise center or an organized climate. Recurrence (how frequently), force (how

hard), and time (how long) make the biggest difference.

"Begin where you are and continuously increment your active work," some activity is great yet more is better."

Requiring 10,000 stages a day is a famous objective since research has shown that when joined with other solid ways of behaving, it can prompt a diminishing in constant sicknesses like diabetes, metabolic conditions, and coronary illness. Practice needn't bother with to be finished in continuous

minutes. You can stroll for 30 to an hour one time per day or you can do exercises a few times each day in 10 to brief additions.

5. Oversee glucose levels

For good preventive well-being, cut back on pop, treats, and sweet pastries, which can cause glucose to rise. Assuming you have diabetes, this can harm your heart, kidneys, eyes, and nerves over the long run.

Besides understanding what compels your glucose levels to climb, the American Heart Affiliation suggests eating shrewd, dealing with your weight,

stopping smoking, and moving more as measures to deal with your glucose.

6. Get a serene rest

Rest reestablishes us and massively affects how we feel. If you experience difficulty resting, attempt to lay out a rest schedule. A decent rest routine incorporates hitting the sack awakening simultaneously consistently and trying not to eat weighty dinners and liquor. It's vital to prevent screen time from your gadgets 2 hours before sleep time, as well.

To slow down before bed:

Pay attention to quieting music.
Practice care or reflection.
Ponder the positive snapshots of the day.
Peruse a book.
Have some chamomile tea.
Practice 10 minutes of yoga.
"Research shows that everyday work-out further develops rest in patients with a sleeping disorder as well, attempt to keep away from overwhelming activity 2 to 3 hours before sleep time.

7. Try not to miss wellbeing screenings and immunizations

It's no distortion: wellbeing screenings can save your life. They are intended to get malignant growths and difficult issues ahead of schedule for more effective therapy.

There are evaluating proposals for grown-ups and ladies explicitly, and differed screenings relying upon your family ancestry, some screening suggestions have changed, so converse with your PCP.

Making sound way of life changes, for the time being, isn't reasonable, yet doing whatever it may take to guarantee you're keeping steady over your well-being will put you ahead and assist you with being the best you can be.

Chapter Three

How food can beat sickness in our body framework

At the point when you center around eating an eating regimen wealthy in natural products, vegetables, and entire grains, you're consequently assisting yourself with forestalling a large number of normal sicknesses, including coronary illness, diabetes, and malignant growth, as per the Places for Infectious prevention and Counteraction.

Food supplements help the safe framework in more than one way: filling in as a cancer prevention agent to safeguard sound cells, supporting the development and action of resistant cells, and delivering antibodies. Epidemiological examinations observe that the people who are inadequately sustained are at a more serious gamble of bacterial, viral, and different contaminations.

Consistently, your body makes it workable for you to think, dream, inhale, rest, and move. Getting the right supplements makes it more straightforward for your body to help you.

Legitimate sustenance assists you with warding off disease, assists you with battling all popular and bacterial contaminations all the more successfully, Works on your state of mind and energy level, diminishes nervousness and sorrow, can't fill in for social separating or wearing a veil around others, and be a way of life, as opposed to a severe eating routine or counting calories

Eating food sources that decrease aggravation ("mitigating" food varieties) helps your resistant framework.

At the point when intruders show up, your body conveys a SOS sign to make your invulnerable framework aware of aggravation. Irritation is a sob for help, an official statement of war to sound caution against intruders.

Irritation: Assists your body with killing trespassers, shields you from contamination, closely resembles redness, expanding, intensity, and agony

The body directs irritation through the safe framework. Your insusceptible framework can

sound alert (cause irritation) even without trespassers around.

The most effective method to involve food as medication to forestall, and invert ongoing sicknesses

NEW ORLEANS — Empowering an energizing eating regimen in patients advances the counteraction and inversion of persistent sicknesses, like CVD, diabetes, malignant growth, and weight, as per a show at the ACP Inward Medication Meeting.

"Of the ten driving reasons for death in the US, somewhere around seven, including the best four, are straightforwardly connected with diet decisions," Michelle McMacken, MD, right-hand teacher of medication at New York College Institute of Medication, said during her show.

These circumstances incorporate coronary illness, malignant growth, lung sickness, cerebrovascular infection, Alzheimer's, diabetes, and kidney illness, as indicated by McMacken.

Force of Sustenance

Almost 50% of all passings because of coronary illness, stroke, and diabetes are because of poor, less than ideal eating regimen," she said: misguided judgments set up for where the patient is going, McMacken said. She noticed that doctors ought to talk about food sources, not supplements.

Doctors can then assist patients with laying out a particular objective and let them set the rhythm of progress, she said. At follow-up visits, doctors ought to expand on objectives, distinguish what worked, what didn't, and why, put forth new objectives offer help and sympathy, and build up the positive.

It is vital not to have your patients or even yourself depend just on determination," she said. At times it is important to change the climate and routine and structure new propensities, she said.

Doctors ought to include their patients' families to get everybody in total agreement, she said.

"Nobody will be ready to change to a restorative eating routine short-term so arranging feasts and shopping for food likewise assume a significant part," as indicated by McMacken.

Food varieties that help your safe framework

1 Attempt new veggies and natural products. Explicit veggies and natural products that decrease irritation are apples, berries, tomatoes, celery, and onions.

2 Add aged food sources. Aged food sources have "great microbes," a.k.a. probiotics that help your resistant framework. Eating more mature food sources additionally diminishes gas, bulging, and runs. Sauerkraut, yogurt, and fermented tea are extraordinary wellsprings of these strong organisms.

3 Hydrate. Water helps your body normally eliminate poisons and conveys oxygen to your whole body. You don't need to hydrate a day to see a distinction in your well-being. Some additional hydration consistently helps a great deal.

4 Get some omega-3s. Salmon, pecans, and chia seeds have omega-3 unsaturated fats, which diminish irritation. These omega-3s are additionally

ideally suited for development. While making new safeguards, your body involves omega-3s as fundamental "building blocks" in cell walls.

Food sources to stay away from to feel your best

1 Cutoff handled food sources. Pungent, handled food varieties can restrict your body's capacity to successfully battle irresistible sicknesses. Take a stab at downsizing only a tad - supplant chips with carrots for a crunchy nibble.

2 Limit sugar. Sugar is alright with some restraint, however an excess of sugar might debilitate your insusceptible framework.

3 Decline high-fat food varieties. Your stomach could do without a ton of red meat or greasy food varieties, the strong microorganisms in your stomach favor mixed greens, fiber, and other supplement-thick food sources that are simpler to separate.

The type of food you eat will affect your general health: Pick Food varieties that Lift Insusceptibility and Battle Disease
L-ascorbic acid - Citrus Natural products and Greens.
Beta-Carotene - Root Vegetables and Greens.
Vitamin E - Greens, Nuts, and Seeds.
Cancer prevention agents - Green Tea.
Vitamin D - Daylight, Fish and Eggs.
Probiotics, Stomach Wellbeing, and Invulnerability.
Garlic - White blood cell Supporter.
Could supplements forestall viral and bacterial contaminations?
No single food, supplement, or enhancement can forestall contaminations, yet practicing good eating habits assists your body in battling infection. Everything no doubt revolves around balance. Supplements (like nutrients and minerals) can be

useful, however, provided that you're not getting enough of those supplements routinely.
Enhancements can be awful for you if you require some investment. Everything is best with some restraint. Assuming you have hidden or ongoing

medical issues, check with your essential consideration supplier before taking them.

Chapter Four

What food means for wellbeing

The food varieties you eat help your resistant framework. Irritation is a characteristic caution to battle trespassers. However, assuming that it continues excessively lengthy, it can hurt you and your capacity to battle illness.

Food sources to assist you with lessening irritation include:

Apples, berries, tomatoes, celery, and onions (veggies and organic products)

Yogurt, sauerkraut and fermented tea (probiotics)

Salmon, pecans, and chia seeds (omega-3 unsaturated fats)

Regardless of your shape or size, your body is wonderful. It's alright if you've been eating more solace food than expected. Check whether there are ways of blending these intruder-battling food sources into your way of life.

An extraordinary initial step would add a couple of new food varieties to your shopping list.
Every week, we're zeroing in on one of the three support points to work on your general well-being and back your resistant framework.
Rest was the primary mainstay of wellbeing
Food is our second mainstay of well-being for a solid safe framework
Practice is the third mainstay of wellbeing in assisting your body with battling sickness.

Key realities as per WHO: Sanitation, nourishment, and food security are inseparably connected.
An expected 600 million - very nearly 1 out of 10 individuals on the planet - become sick in the wake of eating sullied food and 420 000 kick the bucket consistently, bringing about the deficiency of 33 million sound life years (DALYs).

US$ 110 billion is lost every year in efficiency and clinical costs coming about because of perilous food in low-and center pay nations.

Kids under 5 years old convey 40% of the foodborne sickness trouble, with 125,000 passings consistently. Foodborne infections block financial improvement by stressing medical care frameworks and hurting public economies, the travel industry, and exchange.

Outline

Admittance to adequate measures of protected and nutritious food is vital to supporting life and advancing great well-being.

Dangerous food containing hurtful microbes, infections, parasites, or synthetic substances causes more than 200 sicknesses, going from loose bowels to disease.

It likewise makes an endless loop of infection and hunger, especially influencing babies, small kids, the old, and the debilitated.

The great coordinated effort between state-run administrations, makers, and buyers is expected to assist with guaranteeing sanitation and more grounded food frameworks.

Major foodborne sicknesses and causes

Foodborne ailments are typically irresistible or harmful and brought about by microbes, infections, parasites, or compound substances entering the body through polluted food.

Compound tainting can prompt intense harming or long-haul infections, like malignant growth. Numerous foodborne infections might prompt enduring handicaps and demise.

A few instances of food risks are recorded below.

Microbes, Salmonella, Campylobacter, and enterohaemorrhagic Escherichia coli are probably the most widely recognized foodborne microbes that influence a great many individuals yearly, in some cases with serious and deadly results.

Food varieties associated with episodes of salmonellosis incorporate eggs, poultry, and different results of creature beginning.

Foodborne instances of Campylobacter are brought about by crude milk, crude or half-cooked poultry, and drinking water.

Enterohaemorrhagic Escherichia coli is related to unpasteurized milk, half-cooked meat, and debased new foods grown from the ground.

Listeria contaminations can prompt unnatural birth cycles in pregnant ladies or the passing of infants. Even though illness events are moderately low, Listeria's extreme and some of the time deadly well-being outcomes, especially among babies, youngsters, and the older, consider them a real part of the most serious foodborne contaminations.

Listeria is tracked down in unpasteurized dairy items and different prepared-to-eat food varieties and can develop at refrigeration temperatures.

Vibrio cholerae can taint individuals through polluted water or food.

Side effects might incorporate stomach agony, heaving, and lavish watery looseness of the bowels, which rapidly lead to serious drying out and perhaps passing.

Rice, vegetables, millet slop, and different kinds of fish have been embroiled in cholera episodes.

Antimicrobials, like anti-toxins, are vital for treating diseases brought about by microorganisms, including foodborne microbes.

Nonetheless, their abuse and abuse in veterinary and human medication have been connected to the development and spread of safe microorganisms, delivering the treatment of irresistible illnesses insufficient in creatures and people.

Infections

Some infections can be caused by food utilization. Norovirus is a typical reason for foodborne contaminations that are portrayed by sickness, unstable regurgitating, watery runs, and stomach torment.

Hepatitis An infection can likewise be communicated by food and can cause enduring liver sickness and spreads commonly through crude or half-cooked fish or polluted crude produce.

Parasites

A few parasites, for example, fish-borne trematodes, are just sent through food. Others, for instance,

tapeworms like Echinococcus spp, or Taenia spp, may taint individuals through food or direct contact

with creatures. Different parasites, for example, Ascaris, Cryptosporidium, Entamoeba histolytica, or Giardia, enter the established pecking order utilizing water or soil and can debase new produce.

Prions

Prions, irresistible specialists made out of protein, are remarkable in that they are related to explicit types of neurodegenerative illness.

Ox-like spongiform encephalopathy (BSE, or somewhere in the vicinity called distraught cow illness) is a prion sickness in steers, related to the variation Creutzfeldt-Jakob infection (vCJD) in people. Consuming meat items containing determined risk material, for example, cerebrum tissue, is the most probable course of transmission of the prion specialist to people.

Synthetics

Most well-being concerns are normally happening poisons and ecological contaminations.

Normally poisons incorporate mycotoxins, marine biotoxins, cyanogenic glycosides, and poisons found in harmful mushrooms.

Staple food sources like corn or oats can contain elevated degrees of mycotoxins, like aflatoxin and ochratoxin, delivered by old grain.

Long haul openness can influence the resistant framework and typical turn of events, or cause malignant growth.

Steady natural poisons (POPs) are intensified and gather in the climate and the human body.

They are tracked down overall in the climate and collected in creature well-established pecking orders.

Dioxins are profoundly harmful and can create conceptive and formative issues, harm the safe framework, slow down chemicals, and cause malignant growth.

Heavy metals like lead, cadmium, and mercury cause neurological and kidney harm. Tainting by weighty metals in food happens primarily through contamination of water and soil.

Other synthetic perils in food can incorporate radioactive nucleotides that can be released into the climate from businesses and common or military atomic tasks, food allergens, buildups of medications, and different impurities consolidated in the food during the cycle.

Things to be familiar with food illness

What is food illness? Food sickness implies Disease brought about by food sullied with microbes, infections, parasites, or poisons.

Foodborne sickness is brought about by eating sullied food varieties or refreshments.

A wide range of sickness-causing microorganisms or microbes can pollute food sources, so there are various kinds of foodborne diseases.

Most foodborne sicknesses are diseases brought about by different microorganisms, infections, and parasites.

Botulism, Brucellosis, Campylobacter enteritis, Escherichia coli, Hepatitis A, Listeriosis, Salmonellosis, Shigellosis, Toxoplasmosis, Viral gastroenteritis, Taeniasis and Trichinosis are instances of foodborne sicknesses.

What are the normal food sicknesses? As indicated by the CDC, the most widely recognized foodborne diseases are brought about by norovirus, Salmonella, Clostridium perfringens, Campylobacter, and Staphylococcus aureus.

What are the 7 significant foodborne sicknesses?

In any case, the CDC assesses that around 90% of all foodborne sicknesses in this nation are brought about by the accompanying seven (7) microorganisms: Norovirus, Salmonella, Clostridium perfrigens, Campylobacter, Listeria, E. coli 0157:H7 and Toxoplasma.

How might you forestall foodborne sickness?

Forestalling foodborne ailments is a significant general well-being task. The U.S. Branch of Farming and the CDC
Confided in Source have given food handling rules to assist you with trying not to end up being wiped out with a foodborne disease.

They suggest
Cleaning up: Clean up frequently and completely with warm, foamy water for something like 20 seconds when taking care of crude or cooked food varieties, utilizing the washroom, dealing with pets, or keeping an eye on any individual who is sick.

Cleaning things well: Clean food surfaces, utensils, and cutting sheets with hot, sudsy water after each utilization. Figure out how to clean your wooden cutting board.

Isolating food varieties: Keep crude meat, poultry, fish, and eggs separate from cooked and food varieties, including products of the soil, to keep away from cross-tainting.

Preparing food completely: Cook food sources to a safe interior temperature to keep away from half-cooking and lessen foodborne disease risk. Utilize this definite cooking temperature rundown to direct you.

Keeping away from crude refreshments: Try not to drink crude and unpasteurized dairy and juice items.

Putting away food appropriately: Keep food varieties out of the temperature peril zone of 40-140°F (5-60°C) by defrosting frozen food securely in the cooler and refrigerating food varieties in no less than 2 hours of cooking.

If you're debilitated: Remain at home assuming you're feeling unwell and abstain from getting ready nourishment for others during this time, in any event, for a few days after your side effects have died down to Separate when.

How are foodborne ailments treated?

Treatment for foodborne diseases might include a mix of at-home cures and over-the-counter and doctor-prescribed prescriptions.

Nonetheless, the kinds of drugs that medical care experts recommend will rely upon the sort of microorganism answerable for the foodborne disease and the seriousness of side effects. Extreme cases might require hospitalization.

An advise by medical care proficient was that you: drink additional liquids to remain hydrated on the off chance that you have looseness of the bowels or spewing, get additional rest if you are feeling exhausted, take anti-toxins, whenever recommended accept immunizing agents as controlled think about a medical procedure for a few parasitic and poisonous cases

The primary concern: Foodborne disease can happen if you devour food sources or refreshments tainted with hurtful microorganisms — like microbes, infections, or parasites — or their poisons.

Food contamination is a kind of foodborne sickness brought about by ingesting poisons in food sources. Foodborne ailments might come about because of polishing off crude, half-cooked, or sullied meat, fish, poultry, natural products, vegetables, canned merchandise, or drinking water.

Diseases might be determined inside the space of days or months, contingent upon the sort of microorganism and the seriousness of the ailment. Medical care experts might treat these sicknesses with a blend of at-home cures and over-the-counter or professionally prescribed meds.

You can lessen your possibility of contracting foodborne diseases by cleaning up, food arrangement surfaces, utensils, and cutting sheets frequently with warm, foamy water; isolating crude food sources from cooked food sources; and putting away food sources appropriately.

Summary

A sound eating regimen is an eating routine that keeps up with and works on general speaking well-being. It gives the body fundamental supplements, liquid, macronutrients like protein, macronutrients like nutrients, and satisfactory fiber and food energy. It is important to eat a wide range of sorts of food, such as vegetables, salad, cereals, rice, pasta, potatoes, and pieces of bread, wholegrain renditions of these, milk, yogurt, and cheddar, protein, lean meats and poultry, fish, eggs, beans, and nuts, beans and eggs, low-fat spreads and vegetable oils, and sound tidbits like natural product, vegetables, low-fat dairy, and high-fiber oats rather than snacks high in fat, sugar, and salt like desserts, cakes, and crisps. It is also important to have sound tidbits like natural products, vegetables, low-fat dairy, and high-fiber oats rather than snacks high in fat, sugar, and salt like desserts, cakes, and crisps. Finally, it is important to have sound tidbits like natural products, and vegetables.

The most important details in this text are that quality food is key to well-being and that it can help

the body, cerebrum, and mind. Good food can also help the body in more than one way, such as expanding the creation of new neurons and influencing the synaptic versatility of the mind. Good eating habits can also help with weight upkeep, a superior state of mind, expanded energy levels, positive motivation to other people, and the potential for uplifted personal satisfaction. Research has found that soy food sources can cause a drop in testosterone levels, but other research has found that soy-based food sources don't affect testosterone levels.

The most important details in this text are that sickness is a problem of construction or capability in a human, creature, or plant, particularly one that has a known reason and an unmistakable gathering of side effects, signs, or physical changes. Illness is any condition that breaks down the typical working of parts of the body, like cells, tissues, and organs. It can kill cells and tissues, by and large, create poisons that can deaden, obliterate cells' metabolic hardware, or encourage a monstrous safe response that is itself harmful. Ischemic coronary illness is the main source of death all over the planet, and other circumstances, like stroke, COPD, lower respiratory

diseases, and respiratory malignant growths, also represent a huge part of passings every year. To get away from illness, it is important to stay away from super-handled food varieties and eat custom-made dinners arranged with fundamental fixings. All solid weight control plans share include foods grown from the ground, beans, lentils, entire grains like quinoa, earthy colored rice, steel-cut oats, nuts, etc.

The most important details in this text are that it is important to have your cholesterol checked, watch your circulatory strain, get up and get rolling, cut back on pop, treats, and sweet pastries, get serene rest, and not miss health screenings and immunizations. These measures can help reduce the risk of coronary illness and stroke, which are driving reasons for death in the US. Additionally, it is important to get regular exercise, cut back on pop, treats, and sweet pastries, get serene rest, and not miss health screenings and immunizations. Finally, it is important to make sound way of life changes for the time being, but doing whatever it takes to ensure you are keeping steady over your well-being will put you ahead and help you to become the best version of yourself.

The most important details in this text are that eating an eating regimen rich in natural products, vegetables, and entire grains can help to prevent several common illnesses, including coronary illness, diabetes, and malignant growth. Food supplements help the safe framework in more than one way, filling in as a cancer prevention agent to safeguard sound cells, supporting the development and action of resistant cells, and delivering antibodies.

Epidemiological examinations observe that the people who are inadequately sustained are at more serious risk of bacterial, viral, and different contaminations. Doctors should talk about food sources, not supplements, and help patients with laying out a particular objective and setting the rhythm of progress. At follow-up visits, doctors should expand on objectives, distinguish what worked, what didn't, and why, put forth new objectives, offer help and sympathy, and build up the positive. It is important to change the climate and routine and structure new propensities, and doctors should include their patients' families to get everybody in total agreement.

The most important details in this text are the three mainstays of well-being for a strong safe framework: rest, food, and practice. Rest is the primary mainstay of well-being, while food is the second mainstay of well-being, and practice is the third mainstay of well-being. Eating new veggies and natural products, adding aged food sources, hydrating, and getting some omega-3s are all important for a strong safe framework. To feel your best, cut handled food sources, limit sugar, and decline high-fat food varieties. Supplements can be useful, but practicing good eating habits assists your body in battling infection. Food varieties that help your resistant framework include apples, berries, tomatoes, celery, onions, yogurt, sauerkraut, fermented tea, salmon, pecans, chia seeds, mixed greens, fiber, and other supplement thick food sources that are easier to separate. Regardless of your shape or size, your body is wonderful, so check whether there are ways of blending these intruder-battling food sources into your way of life.

The World Health Organization (WHO) estimates that 600 million people become sick in the wake of eating sullied food and 420,000 kick the bucket annually, resulting in the deficiency of 33 million

sound life years (DALYs). US\$ 110 billion is lost every year in efficiency and clinical costs coming about because of perilous food in low-and center pay nations. Foodborne ailments are typically irresistible or harmful and caused by microbes, infections, parasites, or compound substances entering the body through polluted food. Antimicrobials, like anti-toxins, are vital for treating diseases brought about by microorganisms, including foodborne microbes, but their abuse and abuse in veterinary and human medication have been connected to the development and spread of safe microorganisms, delivering the treatment of irresistible illnesses insufficient in creatures and people. Parasites, such as fish-borne trematodes, tapeworms, and parasites, can taint individuals through food or direct contact with creatures and can debase new produce. Prions, such as coccidiosis, Prions are irresistible specialists made out of protein that are related to specific types of neurodegenerative illness. Ox-like spongiform encephalopathy (BSE) is a prion sickness in steers, related to the variation of Creutzfeldt-Jakob infection (vCJD) in people. Synthetic perils include mycotoxins, marine biotoxins, cyanogenic

glycosides, and poisons found in harmful mushrooms. Heavy metals like lead, cadmium, and mercury cause neurological and kidney harm. Other synthetic perils in food can include radioactive nucleotides, food allergens, buildups of medications, and different impurities consolidated in the food during the cycle. Food illness is a disease brought about by food sullied with microbes, infections, parasites, or poisons. The most widely recognized foodborne diseases are brought about by norovirus, salmonella, Clostridium perfringens, Campylobacter enteritis, Escherichia coli, Hepatitis A, Listeriosis, and Salmonellosis.

www.ingramcontent.com/pod-product-compliance
Lightning Source LLC
Chambersburg PA
CBHW070735260726
48660CB00007B/2864